Wound Care Pocket Guide

Myrna Jamont,
RN IIWCC

Published by:

FriesenPress

Suite 300 – 852 Fort Street
Victoria, BC, Canada V8W 1H8

www.friesenpress.com

Distributed to the trade by The Ingram Book Company

Any procedure described in this booklet should be applied by the health care practitioner in accordance with professional standards of care used with regard to the unique circumstances that apply in each practice situation.

No part of this book may be reproduced in any form or by any means without written permission from the owner.

The Pocket Guide is NOT INTENDED to serve as a primary text from which to learn wound care. It's detail is insufficient for these purposes. It is intended instead as a mechanism for review and recall and a convenient, brief, and portable reference.

TABLE OF CONTENTS

To view images online visit:

Pressure ulcers: http://www.npuap.org/
"Reproduction of the National Pressure Ulcer Advisory Panel."

Leg Ulcers: www.legulcerforum.org/imagebanks/view?b

Diabetic Foot: do an online search of *'images for photos of diabetic feet'* in your web browser.

For more information:

DIABETIC FOOT
For plantar pressure redistribution information, please see page 26 of the following paper:

Botros M, et al. Best practice recommendations for the prevention, diagnosis and treatment of diabetic foot ulcers: Update 2010. Wound Care Canada. 2010;6(4):6-40. Available at: http://cawc.net/images/uploads/wcc/8-4-DFU%20BP.pdf.

INLOW TOOL
To access Inlow's 60-Second Diabetic Foot Screen Screening Tool, please visit: http://cawc.net/images/uploads//CAWC_Foot_Ulcer_Screen_Tool_3pg_101E.pdf.

MATERIAL FROM VENOUS LEG ULCER BPR
Reprinted with permission from: Burrows C, et al. Best practice recommendations for the prevention and treatment of venous leg ulcers: Update 2006. Wound Care Canada. 2006;4(1):45-55. Available at: http://cawc.net/images/uploads/wcc/4-1-vol4no1-BP-VLU.pdf.

CLINICAL WOUND ASSESSMENT

Assess and develop a patient care plan:

1. history - comorbidities
2. etiology - cause/origin of wound determined by medical diagnosis
3. environment - home/institution
4. patient and caregiver support - ensure monitoring procedures are understood and followed
5. wound aspect - e.g. location, size, depth, undermining, exudate
6. conditions that may affect healing- e.g. nutritional status, diabetes
7. wound base e.g. if wound base is 100% beefy red choose a different product than 10% red, 90% yellow slough

Principals of care

1. cleanse the wound, debride necrotic tissue
2. control infection
3. fill dead space
4. balance moisture e.g. hydrogels for dry wound , alginates for high exudating wounds
5. address the cause

Adapted with permission from : Wound Assessment and Documentation by Lia van Rijswijk. In :Krasner D, Rodeheaver G, Sibbald RG ,editors. Chronic wound care : a clinical source book for healthcare professionals.3rd ed. Wayne(PA): HMP Comunnications;2001.p103

Phase

1	Hemostasis	Immediate response Cessation of bleeding (clot formation)
2	Inflammation	Control infection (0-4 days) Release growth factors
3	Proliferation	(4 -21 days) Collagen production Granulation Re-epithelialization Contracture
4	Maturation	(Up to 2 years) Remodeling

Adapted with permission from: Chronic Wound Healing and Chronic Wound Management by Dr. Dean Kane.

In : Krasner D, Rodeheaver G, Sibbald RG, editors.Chronic Wound Care :a sourcebook for health care professionals. 3rd ed.Wayne (PA):HMP Comunications; 2001. p 13

Wound Care Management

Complete a wound care record on initial assessment. Reassess wound on each visit to decide appropriate intervention. eg. too wet, too dry, increased exudate.
Pressure Ulcer Record eg. Bates Jensen Wound Assessment Tool (Appendix A)
Lower Limb Record eg. LUMT (Appendix B)
Diabetic Foot Screen (Appendix D)

Note: A wound that is not 30% smaller by week 4 is unlikely to heal by week 12. If an ulcer is not progressing in a measurable way, several items must be reassessed: the treatment, the cause, local wound care, and client-related issues.

Manage pain - pretreatment.

Wound Cleansing

1. Cleanse with warm saline initially and at each dressing change.

2. Irrigate with pressure ranges between 4 and 15 psi. eg.:
    • 35 milliliter syringe with a 19 gauge angiocath, or
    • single-use 100 milliliter saline squeeze bottle.

3. Contraindicated for clients with a ABPI of <0.5. Treat by drying out wound with betadine or cicatrin powder.

4. Do not use <u>antiseptic</u> agents (eg., povidone iodine, iodophor, sodium hypochlorite solution (Dakin's), hydrogen peroxide (acetic acid) to clean wounds with healthy granulating tissue.

Debridement

1. Sharp - for urgent need of debridement. eg. cellulitis or sepsis

   Note: *This procedure requires* **specialized training** *for nurses. Sharp Debridement is a high-risk procedure.*

2. Mechanical - force used to remove non-viable debris. eg. wound irrigation

3. Enzymatic - applying enzymes to necrotic tissue. eg. santyl

4. Autolytic - action of the enzymes in wound fluids eg. hydrocolloids

5. Vascular assessment - recommended for ulcers in lower extremities prior to debridement.

6. Foot ulcers with dry eschar need not be debrided, trim off detached/loose peripheral fragments. Any debridement beyond this can lead to further eschar formation and if debridement is repeated, the wound will gradually deepen, and will ultimately end in bone exposure.

Dressings

Change dressings based on an assessment of the patient and wound, not on routines.

1. Moisture balance
    1) in excessively moist wound, reduce the moisture eg. by using Mepilex Transfer, secondary absorption, an evaporative cover dressing
    2) maintain wounds of arterial etiology where the goal is to dry out the wound

2. Criteria for dressing:
    • controls exudate, keeping the wound bed moist and periwound dry;
    • thermal insulation;
    • protects from contamination;
    • does not leave fibers within wound;
    • no trauma on removal;
    • use sacral-shaped dressings near anus.

3. Use active wound therapies e.g. (biological agents, skin grafts, adjunctive therapies when healing has not progressed)

Infection

1. All open pressure ulcers are colonized with bacteria. Foul odour after thorough cleansing is the only odour that is significant.

2. Signs and symptoms:
    (a) increasing bioburden:
    redness, heat , edema, purulent drainage, foul odour and pain;
    (b) infection:
    Systemic: fever (>38° C), increased pulse, hypotension, mental confusion, agitation, general malaise (blood culture is done to identify organisms). Systemic response requires antibiotic.

    Note: Clients may not show signs of infection if they are immune suppressed, diabetic, elderly, or on steroids.

3. Antibiotics should be effective against gram-negative, gram-positive and anaerobic organisms.

4. Systemic antibiotic therapy for patients with bacteremia, sepsis, cellulitis, or osteomyelitis.

5. Treatment options for bacterial overgrowth:
    - Anti-microbial dressings
    - Dakins, iodine solutions and silver nitrate.

6. Reassess treatment plan with physician every two weeks or as necessary if redness, bleeding and pain occur.

7. To obtain a swab, cleanse wound with saline. With firm pressure, rotate swab in wound bed (not touching exudate, eschar or edges.)

Pressure Ulcer Risk Assessment and Management Algorithm

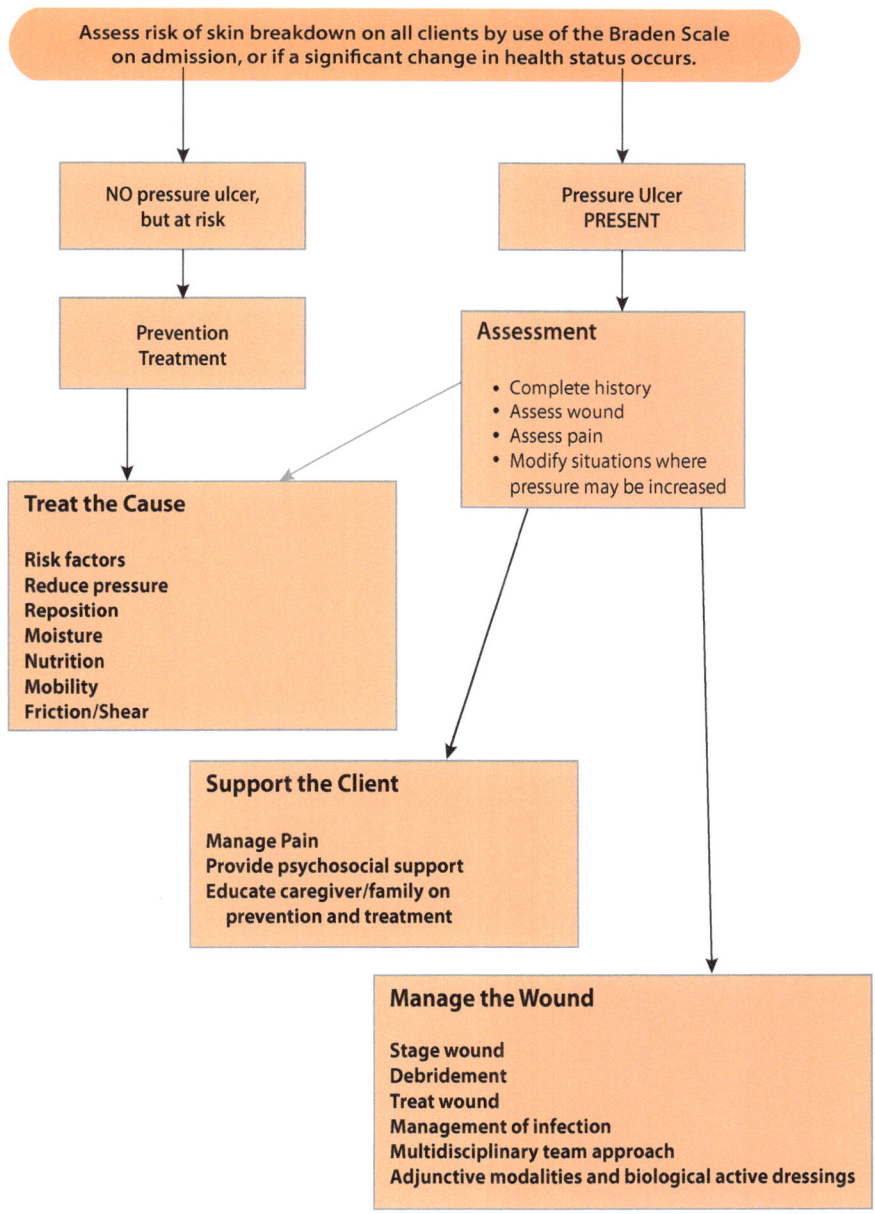

Assess risk of skin breakdown on all clients by use of the Braden Scale on admission, or if a significant change in health status occurs.

NO pressure ulcer, but at risk

Pressure Ulcer PRESENT

Prevention Treatment

Assessment

- Complete history
- Assess wound
- Assess pain
- Modify situations where pressure may be increased

Treat the Cause

**Risk factors
Reduce pressure
Reposition
Moisture
Nutrition
Mobility
Friction/Shear**

Support the Client

**Manage Pain
Provide psychosocial support
Educate caregiver/family on
    prevention and treatment**

Manage the Wound

**Stage wound
Debridement
Treat wound
Management of infection
Multidisciplinary team approach
Adjunctive modalities and biological active dressings**

**For clinical decisions on pressure ulcers use the Braden Scale.
(Appendix C)**

Pressure Ulcers

Non-blanchable erythema of intact skin not resolving within 30 minutes of reducing the cause (pressure). Usually over bony prominence. The area may be painful, firm, soft, warmer or cooler.

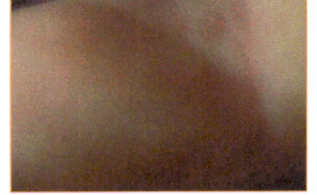

Position the patient off the affected area.

Treatment A

1. Apply moisturizing cream.
2. Avoid massaging.

Treatment B

1. Apply skin barrier/sealant.
2. Apply film dressing.

Stage II

Partial thickness skin loss involving epidermis, dermis or both. The ulcer is superficial and presents clinically as an abrasion, blister or crater. This stage should not be used to describe skin tears, tape burns, perineal dermatitis, maceration or excoriation.

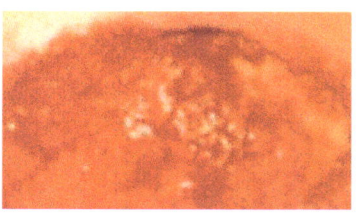

1. ***Position the patient off the affected area.***
2. Cleanse with saline.

Treatment A - Stage II Blister

- Apply transparent film dressing with 2" (5 cm) margin around wound.
- Change if blister fluid has been re-absorbed, or blister is leaking.

Treatment B - Stage II Abrasion or shallow crater

- Apply a skin barrier/sealant to periwound skin.
- Apply hydrocolloid or adhesive foam dressing.

Stage III

Full thickness skin loss involving damage to, or necrosis of, extend down to, but not through underlying fascia. May include undermining and tunneling. Slough may be present.

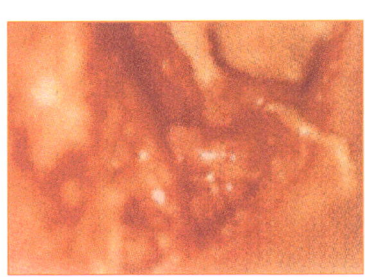

1. ***Position the patient off the affected area.***
2. Cleanse with saline.
3. Remove slough/necrosis.
4. Apply skin barrier/sealant to periwound.
5. Apply topical antimicrobial*.

Treatment A - Stage III with moderate to heavy exudate

- Place an alginate in wound.
- Cover with a high-absorbency/foam dressing.

Treatment B - Stage III without necrosis, minimal exudate.

- Apply thin layer of hydrogel to wound bed.
- Cover with light absorbent dressing.

Stage IV

Full thickness tissue loss with exposed bone, tendon or muscle. Slough or eschar may be present. Often include undermining and tunneling.

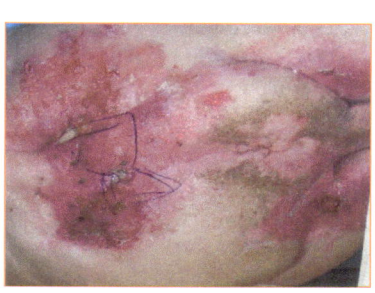

Possible deep cavity with moderate to heavy exudate.

1. *Position the patient off the affected area.*
2. Cleanse with saline. Remove slough/eschar.
3. Apply a topical antimicrobial*.
4. Apply skin barrier/sealant to periwound.
5. Place alginate or cavity dressing in wound.
6. Cover with high absorbency/foam dressing.

* Topical antibiotics such as bacitracin, neomycin, polymyxin B, gentamicin, silver sulfadiazine, erythromycin, and pseudomonic acid (mupirocin) may be used. However, contact dermatitis, anaphylaxis, systemic absorption, toxicity, and bacterial resistance may occur. Therefore, topical antibiotics should be limited to non-healing ulcers and used for 2 weeks or less. **Consult a doctor before applying topical antibiotics.**

Full thickness tissue loss covered by slough or eschar. Remove slough and eschar to expose the base of the wound to determine the depth and stage of wound.

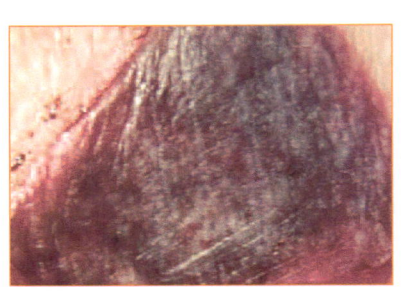

1. ***Position the patient off the affected area.***
2. Cleanse wound with saline. Remove slough/eschar. (Removal of eschar does not apply to black eschar on toes or heels.)
3. Apply a topical antimicrobial*.
4. Apply skin barrier/sealant to periwound.
5. Loosely pack with cavity dressing.
6. Cover with high absorbency/foam dressing.

* Topical antibiotics such as bacitracin, neomycin, polymyxin B, gentamicin, silver sulfadiazine, erythromycin, and pseudomonic acid (mupirocin) may be used. However, contact dermatitis, anaphylaxis, systemic absorption, toxicity, and bacterial resistance may occur. Therefore, topical antibiotics should be limited to non-healing ulcers and used for 2 weeks or less. **Consult a doctor before applying topical antibiotics.**

Deep Tissue Injury

Purple or maroon localized area of discolored intact skin or blood-filled blister due to damage of underlying soft tissue from pressure and/or shear. The area may be painful, firm, mushy, boggy, warm or cool.

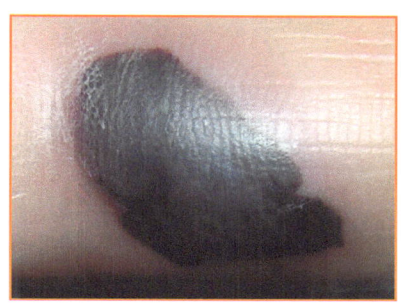

Position the patient off the affected area.

These injuries are to be assessed and treatment individually planned for each case.

The NPUAP states that reverse staging does not accurately characterize what is lost muscle. When ulcers heal to more shallow depth, lost muscle, subcutaneous fat, and dermis does not re-epithelialize. To illustrate: a Stage IV ulcer cannot become a Stage III, Stage II and/or a Stage I ulcer.

Scar tissue is at increased risk of re-ulceration because it will not achieve greater than 80% of the pre-injury tensile strength.

LOWER LIMB ULCERS

ASSESSMENT
1. complete history
2. wound assessment
3. vascular assessment (ABPI)
4. investigations

TREAT THE CAUSE FOR ANY TYPE OF ULCER
- vascular flow
- ankle joint mobility
- venous reflux

Client Concerns
- pain
- education for client and family
- emotional support

Treat the Wound
- moisture balance
- treat infection
- avoid moist wound healing if inadequate blood
  supply to heal wound
- appropriate adjunctive therapies

VENOUS STASIS ULCERS

a. situated on gaiter area of leg
b. shallow, moist wound
c. peri-wound may have maceration or dermatitis
d. edema
e. in wound bed, may have granulation tissue
   or yellow slough
f. varicose viens
h. hyperpigmentation
i. ankle flare
j. lipodermatosclerosis
k. atrophe blanche

1. punched out appearance
2. shiny, taut skin
3. usually on bony prominence
4. feet cool
5. pulse weak
6. wound bed pale, dry
7. toenails thickened
8. gangrenous toes
9. lack of hair on legs & feet
10. dependent rubor

Elastic Systems

Pressure	Characteristics	Examples
Low	Single layer	Comprilan™
High	Long stretch	Surepress™
High	Four layer	Profore™

Inelastic Systems

Pressure	Characteristics	Examples
Low	Flexible cohesive + padding*	Coban™ + cast padding Rolflex™
Low	Zinc oxide bandage + gauze	Unna's Paste Boot
Moderate	Zinc oxide bandage +/- gauze + cohesive	Modified Duke Boot (Viscopate™ + Coban™)
Moderate	Velcro system	Circaid™
Moderate to High	Short-stretch system	Comprilan™

* While cohesive bandages do have some stretch they are best considered to be inelastic systems.

* Reprinted with permission from: Burrows C, et al.

Saskatchewan uses Coban 2 compression therapy.

Obtaining an Ankle-brachial Pressure Index (ABPI)

- The patient is required to lie in the supine position for 15 minutes.
- Brachial blood pressures are obtained in both arms, and the higher of the two systolic pressures is used.
- Place the blood pressure cuff around the ankle above the malleoli.
- Apply ultrasound gel over the dorsum of the foot to obtain a dorsalis pulse, and at the notch below the medial malleolus to obtain the posterior tibial pulse.
- Place the probe at a 450 angle and obtain an audible pulse.
- Inflate the sphygmomanometer until the pulse is obliterated.
- Slowly release the cuff until the pulse is heard. Use the highest reading of the two pulses (dorsalis pedis and posterior tibial) on each leg for the ankle pressure.
- Divide the ankle systolic pressure by the brachial systolic pressure.
- This number is the ABPI.

$$\frac{\text{ankle systolic pressure}}{\text{brachial systolic pressure}} = ABPI \qquad \frac{100 \ (\text{ankle})}{140 \ (\text{brachial})} = 0.71 \ ABPI$$

Interpretation of ABPI
- > 0.9-1.2 ....normal (1.2 or > should indicate calcification)
- 0.80-0.9 ......mild ischemia (inflow disease may be present)
- 0.50-0.79 ....moderate ischemia
- 0.35-0.49 ....moderately severe ischemia
- 0.20-0.34 ....severe ischemia
- < 0.20 ....likely critical ischemia, but absolute pressure and clinical picture must be considered.

> - **ABPI testing should be performed by trained personnel.**
> - **ABPIs may be falsely elevated in persons with diabetes.**

*Reprinted with permission from: Burrows C, et al.

Tensor bandages and anti-embolic stockings do not provide compression for treatment of venous stasis disease.

1. Graduated compression hosiery - prescribed by physician (at mmHg) and prescribed for life.

2. Venous eczema's main treatment is graduated compression. Eczema resolves with a healing wound and reduced exudate.

3. Treat infection before using compression therapy.

4. Application of high compression therapy should be done by trained practitioner.

5. High compression is more effective than low compression in healing venous ulcers and abcense of arterial disease.

6. Use only where ABPI >0.8.

7. Ankle circumference must be equal to or more than 18 cm when using "high compression".

8. Venous ulcers should be treated with high compression to achieve pressure between 35-40 Hg at the ankle, graduating to half at the calf in the normally shaped limb, as per La Place's Law.

$$P \text{ (sub-bandage pressure)} = \frac{N \text{ (number of layers)} \times T \text{ (tension)} \times C \text{ (a constant)}}{C \text{ (limb circumference)} \times W \text{ (width of bandage)}}$$

DIABETIC FOOT ULCERS

Assessment

1. History
    - comorbidities
    - glycemic control
    - bony /structural deformities
    - vascular status (ABI)
    - footwear & sensation

2. Referral to a podiatrist, orthopaedic surgeon, or vascular surgeon for guidelines to diabetic wound assessment and treatment characteristics.

Provide pressure **Offloading** to reduce pressure even while waiting for specialist assessment.

Provide Wound Care

1 . Cleansing

2 . Debridement
   Debride only when adequate blood supply.

   Use vascular assessment prior to procedure.

   - Sharp debridement if urgent

   - Surgical debridement(including bone & joint resection) (These procedures should be performed by a physician or specially trained health professional.)

   - Autolytic

   - Mechanical

3. Presence of pain in a previously insensate foot can be 1st indicator of infection.

4. Dressings, manage exudate (moisture balance)

5. Consider biological agents & adjunct therapies

Address client concerns

Empower an Interprofessional Teamwork Approach for the following:

- pain

- exercise, ROM

- skin care

- elevate legs

- foot care

- nutrition

- compliance

- emotional concerns

- family & client education

Complete a diabetic foot screen initially and on each consecutive visit.
Appendix D

General Information for Diabetic

Wound Type	Description	Character
Post-surgical	Approximated	Moist
Dry stable eschar or toe gangrene	Necrotic	Dry/black or grey
Necrotic tissue in situ	Necrotic Sloughy	Dry/black or grey Moist/yellow or gray Maladorous
Clean Wound	Granulating	Granulating (red base) Moist May bleed easily

Foot Ulcer Dressing Choices

Bacterial Profile	Blood Supply	Dressing Choices
Sterile	Adequate	Gauze, foam, hydrofiber (depends on amount of exudate)
Colonized ? Infected	Inadequate	Dry out the wound. Betadine, cicatrin, gauze
Colonized ? Infected	Adequate	Debriding products Iodine dressings (Cadexomer / Inadine) depending on moisture level. If largely exudating, hydrofiber and/or foams may be used to control drainage.
Contaminated or colonized	Adequate	Heavily exudating - hydrofibers or alginates, combined with foams, combination products. Moderately exudating - formas +/- hydrofiber (depends on length of wear time) Lightly exudating - thin foams. Wounds in depth fill with ribbon gauze, hydrofibre or alginate.

* Adapted with permission from Revision of the Saskatchewan working group for the Clinical Practice Guidelines for Prevention and Management of Diabetes Foot Complications.

Appendix A

BATES-JENSEN WOUND ASSESSMENT TOOL   NAME _____

Complete the rating sheet to assess wound status. Evaluate each item by picking the response that best describes the wound and entering the score in the item score column for the appropriate date.

Location: Anatomic site. Circle, identify right **(R)** or left **(L)** and use **"X"** to mark site on body diagrams:

____ Sacrum & coccyx   ____ Lateral ankle
____ Trochanter   ____ Medial ankle
____ Ischial tuberosity   ____ Heel   Other Site

Shape: Overall wound pattern; assess by observing perimeter and depth.

Circle and <u>date</u> appropriate description:

____ Irregular   ____ Linear or elongated
____ Round/oval   ____ Bowl/boat
____ Square/rectangle   ____ Butterfly   Other Shape

Item	Assessment	Date Score	Date Score	Date Score
1. Size	1 = Length x width <4 sq cm 2 = Length x width 4--<16 sq cm 3 = Length x width 16.1--<36 sq cm 4 = Length x width 36.1--<80 sq cm 5 = Length x width >80 sq cm			
2. Depth	1 = Non-blanchable erythema on intact skin 2 = Partial thickness skin loss involving epidermis &/or dermis 3 = Full thickness skin loss involving damage or necrosis of subcutaneous tissue; may extend down to but not through underlying fascia; &/or mixed partial & full thickness &/or tissue layers obscured by granulation tissue 4 = Obscured by necrosis 5 = Full thickness skin loss with extensive destruction, tissue necrosis or damage to muscle, bone or supporting structures			
3. Edges	1 = Indistinct, diffuse, none clearly visible 2 = Distinct, outline clearly visible, attached, even with wound base 3 = Well-defined, not attached to wound base 4 = Well-defined, not attached to base, rolled under, thickened 5 = Well-defined, fibrotic, scarred or hyperkeratotic			
4. Under-mining	1 = None present 2 =Undermining < 2 cm in any area 3 = Undermining 2-4 cm involving < 50% wound margins 4 = Undermining 2-4 cm involving > 50% wound margins 5 = Undermining > 4 cm or Tunneling in any area			
5. Necrotic Tissue Type	1 = None visible 2 = White/grey non-viable tissue &/or non-adherent yellow slough 3 = Loosely adherent yellow slough 4 = Adherent, soft, black eschar 5 = Firmly adherent, hard, black eschar			
6. Necrotic Tissue Amount	1 = None visible 2 = < 25% of wound bed covered 3 = 25% to 50% of wound covered 4 = > 50% and < 75% of wound covered 5 = 75% to 100% of wound covered			

Saskatchewan Skin and Wound Care Guidelines, March 2006

24

Item	Assessment	Date Score	Date Score	Date Score
7. Exudate Type	1 = None 2 = Bloody 3 = Serosanguineous: thin, watery, pale red/pink 4 = Serous: thin, watery, clear 5 = Purulent: thin or thick, opaque, tan/yellow, with or without odour			
8. Exudate Amount	1 = None, dry wound 2 = Scant, wound moist but no observable exudate 3 = Small 4 = Moderate 5 = Large			
9. Skin Color Surrounding Wound	1 = Pink or normal for ethnic group 2 = Bright red &/or blanches to touch 3 = White or grey pallor or hypopigmented 4 = Dark red or purple &/or non-blanchable 5 = Black or hyperpigmented			
10. Peripheral Tissue Edema	1 = No swelling or edema 2 = Non-pitting edema extends < 4 cm around wound 3 = Non-pitting edema extends $\geq$ 4 cm around wound 4 = Pitting edema extends < 4 cm around wound 5 = Crepitus and/or pitting edema extends $\geq$ 4 cm around wound			
11. Peripheral Tissue Induration	1 = None present 2 = Induration, < 2 cm around wound 3 = Induration 2-4 cm extending < 50% around wound 4 = Induration 2-4 cm extending $\geq$ 50% around wound 5 = Induration > 4 cm in any area around wound			
12. Granulation Tissue	1 = Skin intact or partial thickness wound 2 = Bright, beefy red; 75% to 100% of wound filled &/or tissue overgrowth 3 = Bright, beefy red; < 75% & > 25% of wound filled 4 = Pink, &/or dull, dusky red &/or fills $\leq$ 25% of wound 5 = No granulation tissue present			
13. Epithelialization	1 = 100% wound covered, surface intact 2 = 75% to < 100% wound covered &/or epithelial tissue extends > 0.5cm into wound bed 3 = 50% to < 75% wound covered &/or epithelial tissue extends to < 0.5cm into wound bed 4 = 25% to < 50% wound covered 5 = < 25% wound covered			
TOTAL SCORE				
SIGNATURE				

WOUND STATUS CONTINUUM

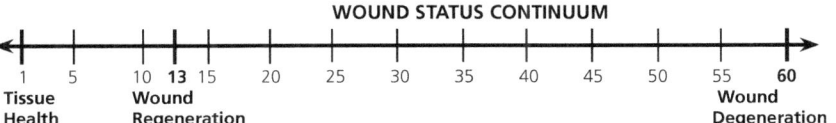

| 1 | 5 | 10 | **13** | 15 | 20 | 25 | 30 | 35 | 40 | 45 | 50 | 55 | **60** |

Tissue Health   Wound Regeneration   Wound Degeneration

Plot the total score on the Wound Status Continuum by putting an "**X**" on the line and the date beneath the line. Plot multiple scores with their dates to see-at-a-glance regeneration or degeneration of the wound.

Printed with permission from: Saskatchewan Skin and Wound Care Guidelines, March 2006.

Appendix B

Leg Ulcer Measurement Tool (LUMT)

© Woodbury, Houghton, Campbell   LUMT 2000.

The Leg Ulcer Measurement Tool (LUMT) must be used without modification and in the manner indicated in the accompanying general instructions.

Item / Domain	Response Categories	Score			
		Date (mm/dd/yyyy)			
		_/_/_ __	_/_/_ __	_/_/_ __	_/_/_ __
(A) CLINICIAN RATED DOMAINS					
A1. Exudate type	**0** None **1** Serosanguinous **2** Serous **3** Seropurulent **4** Purulent				
A2. Exudate amount	**0** None **1** Scant **2** Small **3** Moderate **4** Copious				
A3. Size (from edge of advancing border of epithelium)	**(Length x Width)** **0** Healed **1** <2.5 cm^2 **2** 2.5-5.0 cm^2 **3** 5.1-10.0 cm^2 **4** 10.1 cm^2 or more				
A4. Depth	Tissue Layers **0** Healed **1** Partial thickness skin loss **2** Full thickness **3** Tendon/joint capsule visible **4** Probes to bone				
A5. Undermining	**Greatest at _____ o'clock** **0** 0 cm **1** >0 - 0.4 cm **2** >0.4 - 0.9 cm **3** >0.9 - 1.4 cm **4** >1.5 cm				
A6. Necrotic tissue type	**0** None **1** *Loose* white to yellow slough **2** *Attached* white to yellow slough or fibrin **3** *Soft* grey to black eschar **4** *Hard* dry black eschar				
A7. Necrotic tissue amount	**0** None visible **1** 1 to 25% of wound bed covered **2** 26 to 50% of wound bed covered **3** 51 to 75% of wound bed covered **4** 76 to 100% of wound bed covered				
A8. Granulation tissue type	**0** Healed **1** Bright beefy red **2** Dusky pink **3** Pale **4** Absent				

Item / Domain	Response Categories	Score		
A9. Granulation tissue amount	**0** Healed **1** 76 to 100% of wound bed covered **2** 51 to 75% of wound bed covered **3** 26 to 50% of wound bed covered **4** 1 to 25% of wound bed covered			
A10. Edges	**0** Healed **1** ≥50% advancing border of epithelium or indistinct borders **2** < 50% advancing border of epithelium **3** Attached, no advancing border of epithelium **4** Unattached or undermined			
A11. Periulcer skin viability - callus - dermatitis (pale) - maceration - induration - erythema (bright red) - purple blanchable - purple non-blanchable - skin dehydration	Number of factors affected **0** None **1** One only **2** Two or three **3** Four or five **4** Six or more factors			
A12. Leg edema type	**0** None **1** Non-pitting or firmness **2** Pitting **3** Fibrosis or lipodermatosclerosis **4** Indurated			
A13.Leg edema location	**0** None **1** Localized periulcer **2** Foot, including ankle **3** To mid calf **4** To knee			
A14. Assessment of bioburden	**0** Healed **1** Lightly colonized **2** Heavily colonized **3** Localized infection **4** Systemic infection			
Total - (A) CLINICIAN RATED DOMAINS:				

Item / Domain	Response Categories	Score		
(B) PATIENT (PROXY) RATED DOMAINS				
B1. Pain amount (as it relates to the leg ulcer) *Rate your pain, experienced in the last 24 hours, on a scale from 0 to 10, where 0 is "no pain" and 10 is the "worst pain".*	**Numerical rating scale (0 - 10)** **0** None **1** >0 – 2 **2** >2 – 4 **3** >4 – 7 **4** >7			
B2. Pain frequency (as it relates to the leg ulcer) *"Which of the following terms best describes how often you have had pain in the last 24 hours?"*	**0** None **1** Occasional **2** Position dependent **3** Constant **4** Disturbs sleep			
B3. Quality of life (as it relates to the leg ulcer) *"How do you feel about the quality of your life at the present time?"*	**0** Delighted **1** Satisfied **2** Mixed **3** Dissatisfied **4** Terrible			
Total - (B) PATIENT (PROXY) RATED DOMAINS:				
Proxy Completed by:				
Total LUMT Score:				

Printed with permission from: Saskatchewan Skin and Wound Care Guidelines, March 2006.

Appendix C

Braden Risk Assessment Scale

Note: Bed and chair-bound individuals or those with impaired ability to reposition should be assessed upon admission for their risk of developing pressure ulcers. Patients with established pressure ulcers should be reassessed periodically.

Patient Name: Room Number: Date:

Sensory Perception	1. Completely Limited	2. Very Limited	3. Slightly Limited	4. No Impairment	*Indicate Appropriate Numbers Below*
Ability to respond meaningfully to pressure-related discomfort	Unresponsive (does not moan, flinch or grasp) to painful stimuli, due to diminished level of consciousness or sedation. OR limited ability to feel pain over most of body surface	Responds only to painful stimuli. Cannot communicate discomfort except by moaning or restlessness. OR has a sensory impairment which limits the ability to feel pain or discomfort over $^1/_2$ of body.	Responds to verbal commands, but cannot always communicate discomfort or need to be turned. OR has some sensory impairment which limits ability to feel pain or discomfort in 1 or 2 extremities.	Responds to verbal commands. Has no sensory deficit which would limit ability to feel or voice pain or discomfort.	
Moisture	1. Constantly Moist	2. Very Moist	3. Occasionally Moist	4. Rarely Moist	
Degree to which skin is exposed to moisture.	Skin is kept moist almost constantly by perspiration, urine, etc. Dampness is detected every time patient is moved or turned.	Skin is often, but not always, moist. Linen must be changed at least once a shift.	Skin is occasionally moist, requiring an extra linen change approximately once a day.	Skin is usually dry. Linen only requires changing at routine intervals.	
Activity	1. Bedfast	2. Chair fast	3. Walks Occasionally	4. Walks Frequently	
Degree of physical activity	Confined to bed.	Ability to walk severely limited or non-existent. Cannot bear own weight and/or must be assisted into chair or wheelchair.	Walks occasionally during day, but for very short distances, with or without assistance. Spends majority of each shift in bed or chair.	Walks outside the room at least twice a day and inside room at least once every 2 hours during waking hours.	
Mobility	1. Completely Immobile	2. Very Limited	3. Slightly Limited	4. No limitations	
Ability to change and control body position.	Does not make even slight changes in body or extremity position without assistance.	Makes occasional slight changes in body or extremity position but unable to make frequent or significant change independently.	Makes frequent though slight changes in body or extremity position independently.	Makes major and frequent changes in position without assistance.	
Nutrition	1. Very Poor	2. Probably Inadequate	3. Adequate	4. Excellent	
Usual food intake pattern.	Never eats a complete meal. Rarely eats more than 1/3 of any food offered. Eats 2 servings or less of protein (meat or dairy products) per day. Takes fluids poorly. Does not take a liquid dietary supplement, OR is NPO and/or maintained on clear liquids or I.V.'s for more than 5 days.	Rarely eats a complete meal and generally eats only about $^1/_2$ of any food offered. Protein intake includes only 3 servings of meat or dairy products per day. Occasionally will take a dietary supplement, OR receives less than optimum amount of liquid diet or tube feeding.	Eats over half of most meals. Eats a total of 4 servings of protein (meat, dairy products) each day. Occasionally will refuse a meal, but will usually take a supplement if offered, OR is on tube feeding or TPN regimen which probably meets most of nutritional needs.	Eats most of every meal. Never refuses a meal. Usually eats a total of 4 or more servings of meat and dairy products. Occasionally eats between meals. Does not require supplementation.	
Friction and **Shear**	1. Problem	2. Potential Problem	3. No Apparent Problem		
	Requires moderate to maximum assistance in moving. Complete lifting without sliding against sheets is impossible. Frequently slides down in bed or chair, requiring frequent repositioning with maximum assistance. Spasticity, contractures or agitation lead to almost constant friction.	Moves feebly or requires minimum assistance. During a move, skin probably slides to some extent against sheets, chair restraints, or other devices. Maintains relatively good position in chair or bed most of the time, but occasionally slides down.	Moves in bed and in chair independently and has sufficient muscle strength to lift up completely during move. Maintains good position in bed or chair at all times.		
				Total Score:	

NOTE: Patients with a total score of 16 or less are considered to be at risk of developing pressure ulcers.(15 or 16 = low risk; 13 or 14 = moderate risk; 12 or less = high risk) © Copyright Barbara Braden and Nancy Bergstrom. Used with permission.

Printed with permission from: Saskatchewan Skin and Wound Care Guidelines, March 2006.

Appendix D

Diabetes Foot Screen

Name (Last, First, MI) _____ Date: _____/_____/_____

Fill in the following blanks with a "Y" or "N" to indicate findings in the right or left foot.

	R	L
Is there a history of a foot ulcer?	_____	_____
Is there a foot ulcer now?	_____	_____
Is there a claw toe deformity?	_____	_____
Is there an abnormal foot shape?	_____	_____
Are the toenails, thick or ingrown?	_____	_____
Is there heavy callus build-up?	_____	_____
Is there swelling?		_____
_____ Is there elevated skin temperature?		_____
_____ Is there limited ankle dorsiflexion?		_____
_____ Is there foot or ankle muscle weakness?		_____
_____ Can the patient see the bottom of their feet?		_____
_____ Are the shoes appropriate in style and fit?		_____
_____ Is there an absent pedal pulse?*		_____

Note the level of sensation in the circles:

\+ = Can feel the 5.07 filament   - = Can't feel the 5.07 filament

LEFT   RIGHT

Skin Conditions on the Foot or Between the Toes:

Draw in: Callus ▨,   Pre-ulcer ▦,   Ulcer ■ (note length and width in cm)

Label with: **R** - redness, **M** - maceration, **D** - dryness, **W***- warm **T**-Tinea, **Dis*** - discoloration

RISK CATEGORY:
_____ 0 No loss of protective sensation
_____ 1 Loss of protective sensation
_____ 2 Loss of protective sensation with either high pressure (callus/deformity), or poor circulation
_____ 3 History of plantar ulceration, neuropathic fracture (Charcot foot) or amputation

Rev. 03/22/02 LSUHSC Diabetes Foot Program Performed by: _____

Printed with permission from: Saskatchewan Clinical Practice Guidelines for Prevention and Management of Diabetic Foot Complications, February 2008.

Diabetic Foot Care

Instructions for clients:

DO'S

Wash feet daily in warm water, not hot and do not soak
Dry between toes
Apply lotion to keep skin soft , but not between toes
Change socks daily
Wear shoes and socks all the time. Check nothing is inside shoes
Wear shoes that fit well, with good support and lots of room for toes
Cheek feet daily with a mirror for sores, cracks, and nail problems
Cut toenails straight across
Exercise daily
Schedule regular check-up with nurse ,doctor or foot doctor
Remove socks and shoes to remind them to check feet

DON'TS

Don't walk barefoot indoors or outdoors
Don't go outside in cold weather without warm socks and shoes
Don't get sunburned. Cover feet to protect from sun
Don't cut corns or calluses, have professional person do treatment
Don't use chemicals such as alcohol, peroxide or iodine unless directed by professional
Don't use hot water bottle, or heating pad on your feet
Don't wear tight fitting shoes, sandals or wrinkled socks
Don't cross legs at knees or ankles
Don't leave sores, scrapes or skin cracks unattended. Watch for redness, drainage , warmth and foul odor. Call professional to attend to the problem.
Don't smoke

Adapted from Regina Qu'Appelle Health Region 2008

Dressings for Wounds

PRODUCT	FUNCTIONS
Skin Protectant	
Baza Cleanse & Protect Proshield Plus Remedy	• to moisturize skin and cleanse
Barrier Critic aid clear Sensicare	• eliminates moisture
Skin Sealant Cavilon (No sting wipes & spray) Skin prep All kare Remove	• provides protective barrier (Some contain alcohol. Do not use on open wounds.)
Hydro Gels	
Intrasite Gel Duoderm Gel Tegaderm Gel Nu Gel	• moist wound balance • hydrate eschar and slough • create moisture in dry wound
Non-adhering Dressings	
Mepitel (silicone coated) Adaptic, Digit (*petrolatum*) Bactigras (contains antimicrobial)	• non adherent, non absorbent • open mesh allows exudate to pass vertically onto 2nd dressing
Transparent Films	

OpSite
Tegaderm
	• semi-permeable dressings that are
	  waterproof yet permeable to oxygen and
	  water vapor
	• maintain a moist wound environment

Hydrocolloids	

Comfeel plus transparent
Tegaderm
Combiderm
Restore
	• occlusive
	• react with wound exudate to form a gel-
	  like covering protecting wound bed and
	  maintaining moist environment

INDICATION	ADVANTAGE
• incontinence	• prevent skin breakdown
• adheres to denuded skin	• easy to apply
• to periwound • to enhance adhesion of some covered dressings	• prevents skin irritation • protects from maceration
• donor sites • aiding in natural autolytic process	• effective hydrating • no mixing, preparation • non-adherent; removable without harming granulating tissue
• granulating wounds • skin grafts • skin tears • abrasions and lacerations	• easy to remove with minimum pain and without damaging newly formed granulation tissue
• superficial wounds • covering blisters • to protect skin from feces/urine • facilitate cellular migration	• permits evaluation of wound progress without removal of dressing
• promotes autolytic debridement • for low draining wounds • granulation tissue formation	• waterproof and prevents bacterial and environment contamination

PRODUCT	FUNCTIONS
Alginates	
Tegagen SeaSorb AHL (medihoney) Silvercel NA (sustained silver release)	• composed of alginate fibers & or seaweed • high capacity to absorb wound exudate & creates a soft gel • for packing wounds • hemostatic capabilities
Hydrofiber Dressings	
Aquacel AG Aquacel Surgical Versiva xc	• composed of hydro fiber • highly absorbent of exudate
Impregnated Gauze Dressings	
Mesalt impregnated sodium chloride Viscopaste (zinc coated)	• stimulates the cleansing of wounds • for management of leg ulcers
Charcoal Silver Dressing	
Actisorb with silver	• charcoal adsorbs odour • use on wet or dry wounds • do not cut • requires 2nd dressing
High Absorbency and Foams Dressings	
Mepilex, Lite, Sacrum, Heal, Border Mesorb Biatain Allevyn, Plus Versiva Tegaderm Aquacel Surgical Biatain (ibuprofen)	• high absorbency • excessive wound drainage

INDICATION	ADVANTAGE
• for colonized & infected mod to heavy draining wounds • venous leg ulcers • diabetic foot ulcers • pressure ulcers • trauma • surgical wounds	• conformable to wound shapes • absorbs and retains fluid • decreases frequency of dressing changes
• high exudative chronic wounds and cavities	• absorbs large amounts of exudate • provides moist wound environment
• for infected wounds • leg ulcers • chronic eczema and dermatitis	• stimulates cleansing of wound • easy application
• venous leg ulcers • pressure ulcers • diabetic foot ulcers • fumigating carcinoma • surgical wounds • traumatic wounds	• reduces odor
• exudating wounds • deep cavity wounds • venous leg ulcers	• reduces the number of dressing changes

PRODUCT	FUNCTIONS
Antimicrobial Dressings	
Silvercel Silverlon 100% ionic (roll) (US Military) Aquacel AG Tegaderm AG Arglaes powder Iodosorb (cadexemer iodine) gel, paste Inadine (iodine dressing) Acticoat,Flex3, Flex7 AHL Medihoney	• prevention and treatment of infection • broad spectrum coverage gram +/-, fungi, MRSA, and VRE • 10% povidone iodine has sustained release into wound
Enzymatic/Debrider	
Santyl	• removes necrotic tissue • for wound bed preparation
Collagen Dressings Indicated for chronic wounds free from necrotic tissue & infection.	
Promogran Prisma (silver) Fibracol Plus	• promotes granulation • tissue formation • delivers collagen to wound encouraging proliferation • forms gel on contact with wound fluid
Negative Pressure Wound Therapy	
VAC	• reducing wound margins • encourage granulating tissue

INDICATION	ADVANTAGE
• pressure ulcers • diabetic foot ulcers • leg ulcers • surgical wounds	• decreases bacterial load • broad spectrum • may be used in conjunction with systemic antibiotics • some products may be left on 7 days
• pressure ulcers • venous leg ulcers	• alternative to surgical/sharp debridement
• diabetic ulcers • venous ulcers • pressure ulcers • mixed vascular etiologies • traumatic wounds • surgical wounds	• binds & inactivates excess proteases • bioabsorbable • binds and protects growth factors • compatible with alternative products
• acute • chronic • flaps • trauma • clean, closed incision	• reduces infection • removes fluid from wound

REFERENCES

1. Health Quality Council of Saskatchewan, Saskatchewan Skin and Wound Care Guidelines. March 2006.

2. Saskatchewan working group for the Clinical Practice Guidelines for Prevention and Management of Diabetes Foot Complications. February 2008.

3. Inlow S. A 60 second foot exam for people with diabetes. Wound Care Canada. 2004; 2(2):10-11. CAWC 2010 P1419E

4. Botros M, et al. Best practice recommendations for the prevention, diagnosis and treatment of diabetic foot ulcers: Update 2010. Wound Care Canada.

5. Inlow's 60-Second Diabetic Foot Screen Screening Tool.

6. Burrows C, et al. Best practice recommendations for the prevention and treatment of venous leg ulcers: Update 2006. Wound Care Canada. 2006

7. Wound Assessment and Documentation by Lia van Rijswijk. In: Krasner D, Rodeheaver G, Sibbald RG ,editors. Chronic wound care: a clinical source book for healthcare professionals. 3rd ed. Wayne(PA): HMP Comunnications; 2001.

8. Chronic Wound Healing and Chronic Wound Management by Dr. Dean Kane. In: Krasner D, Rodeheaver G, Sibbald RG, editors. Chronic Wound Care: a source book for health care professionals. 3rd ed. Wayne (PA):HMP Communications; 2001

Myrna Jamont, RN IIWCC

Myrna Jamont, throughout her career, has worked in medicine, surgery, pediatrics and ICU. While employed at a long-term care facility, she became interested in the prevention of skin breakdown and treatment of wounds.

In 2000, she completed the prescribed program of the University of Toronto International Interdisciplinary Wound Care Course.

Her position as Equipment and Standardization Nurse in the Saskatoon Health Region included educating staff on the use of all equipment and products available to prevent and treat wounds.

As a consultant, she continues to educate as a Skin Care and Wound Management Facilitator/Educator.

Acknowledgement
A thank you to Crystal Benoit who added the style and design to this edition.